Toddler S

Proven Methods to Train Your Toddler to Sleep without Getting Frustrated

Table of Contents

Introduction

There are many books that have been written on the subject of training a baby to sleep, but how many of them really tackle the problems from a practical point of view? Some are written by "experts" who haven't even had children let alone really understanding the true nature of the problems faced by parents. What makes this book any different? The fact is that I have brought up more than 5 children but I haven't let my learning be limited to training them. Over the course of years, I have worked with hundreds of babies because of working in the care system and I know that children from all kinds of families have problems that are as varied as the children themselves are. It is my experience in looking after children that prompted me to write this book, from a practical viewpoint, so that parents could relate to the problems that have been addressed within its pages.

Toddlers are at that stage when a child is starting to know what is going on around them. They are aware of bad things and good things and they tend to make their minds up pretty rapidly if they think they are being asked to do something they don't want to do. Unfortunately, many of these little folk have a very powerful position over inexperienced parents. I think that sleep training has to start when the child is a baby, but don't worry if you have not done that yet. I have also told you how to restart the training on your toddler so that you don't have to continue with the battle of wits that happens at bedtime and can indeed let your little monsters get sufficient sleep without even knowing that you are controlling what they do. You have to use child psychology to a certain degree but I want to take the subject back to basics, so that you have a better chance of making bedtime a less traumatic time for everyone.

The child who learns to sleep independently and who is happy to be alone in his bedroom is a child that has the security that every child needs. We see stories of kids who don't have that luxury and when we balance that against the needs of our children, often find ourselves getting angry and frustrated when the toddler has a will of his own and won't do as he/she is bid. Don't worry about that for the time being. By the time you have read this book and understand the way that child sleep patterns are established, you will be well on your way toward letting go of all the worry and knowing that your child is getting the sleep that is needed, at the right time.

The methods described in the book are a mixture of experience and what experts say about sleep as these are people who have studied sleep patterns, and it's important to combine your experience with the experience of experts to get the best results from your sleep training. Your child learns everything that he/she knows from you, and as a parent, it's your responsibility to make sure that the child is sufficiently rested so that the next day is not a battle of wits with a child who is tired and grumpy. Walk through the pages of the book and you will find that gradual changes are occurring and that you are beginning to understand the way it works in real life. Yes, some expert opinions do have merit though they only have merit when they take into consideration your own personal circumstances and your experiences thus far. That's why I wrote this book to fill a gap in the market and to make sure that parents have the best chance possible to get their children to sleep at the right time and for the right number of hours.

Why is sleep so important? We know that sleep is needed for the individual to wake up with sufficient energy to face the next day, but did you know there are also many other benefits to your toddler.

- Sleep is a time of healing and it allows your child to regain physical strength and mental agility
- Sleep allows the child to go through the growing pains smoothly
- Sleep allows you, as a parent to be sufficiently rested to care for your children without losing your temper.
- Sleep benefits children because it helps them to understand the order that life takes
- A child who sleeps well is a healthier and happier child

If you have ever noticed what happens when a toddler gets tired, some of the symptoms of overtiredness include:

- Frayed temper
- Lack of patience
- Unreasonable behavior
- Sleeping during the day

These are all things that you need to put right before your child goes to school. The reason for this is that it benefits the child's learning. If the child is alert and awake during the daytime, it's much more likely that he/she will learn more and be more sociable to other children within the school setting. Therefore, getting it right at an early age is essential.

Join with me through the chapters of this book and learn what it's all about and what you, as a parent, can do to lessen both your stress and the obvious stress of the child. I guarantee that it will work and that you and your child will be a lot happier once you have established a sleep routine that works for both of you. I know that my own experience was enriched by all of the children I have had in my care but I also know that it benefited them too, because I saw the result of happy, balanced and caring children, going into the world with the right attitude and infancy is where it all starts.

By the end of reading this book, you will know what you can do to be happier as a parent and what you need to do to support and love your child sufficiently that he/she sleeps well at night and enjoys the learning experience attached with recognizing the need to sleep.

Chapter One: Gender Differences

One thing that you will notice is that there is a difference in attitude and approach when it comes to the gender of the child. Boys are more difficult to get to go to sleep than girls are and it's by a very high number as well but there are psychological and society reasons why this is so. Girls are quite happy and usually quite cuddly and get a lot of attention from parents. Boys, on the other hand, are usually viewed as more independent because they are boys. Unfortunately, the fact is that boys need cuddles as much as girls do. They are, at this stage, small children, who need the love and support of their parents. There is a very good book that was written by Steve Biddulph called Raising Boys. In it he wrote about the way in which parents see boys and girls as being different entities. We mollycoddle girls in an attempt to protect but when it comes to boys, we tend to see them as being more independent and perhaps don't give them the sense of security that they need to feel.

When you look at premature baby mortality rates, it's very disturbing that boys suffer more than girls do and there's a very good reason for this. Their need to be loved and cuddled is greater than that of their female counterparts. In fact, I remember when one of my kids was born premature, she was in the ICU and the nurses made a point of telling me that I didn't have to worry because girls were much better at coping with the difficulties presented. That thought stayed with me for years as I tried to work out why that was and why boys are so naturally delicate when it comes to sleep patterns.

Up until the age of 3 years old, boys do not have a fully developed brain in the same way as girls do. In fact, girls cope a lot better with the world around them because of this. If you place a girl in a crowded place, she is likely to cope with it more than a boy is. You can almost be certain that the child who is crying for his mother in the store is a boy, rather than a girl, because his brain has not cottoned onto the fact that everything is alright. The slow development of the male brain doesn't mean there is anything wrong, but it does mean that parents need to be aware of the potential of not showing sufficient care when dealing with boys.

From being a baby, a boy needs to be cuddled and to be made to feel secure in the environment he is growing up in. The child's crib may be better in the parent's room, where the child can see his parents. You may find that having a night light also gives that child an extra sense of security. When the child is moved to his own room before the age of three, you are battling with nature. Not only has the child just learned what day and night are about, but he also has to cope with the anxiety of separation that a girl finds easy to cope with. The setting up of the bedroom is of paramount importance and as you will read through in the general instructional part of this book, the child's security should always be borne in mind when dealing with boys under this age.

Post Natal Depression also plays a part in how a baby responds to sleep in the home. Those babies whose mothers suffered from PND were the most difficult to get to sleep. Studies have been done on this to try and find out what the connection is to PND and also to postpartum depression and what seems to be a link is that the child has emotional needs that are not always met by a mother who is going through emotional problems herself and that boys are most likely to suffer worse than girls because their emotional needs are greater than those of their female counterparts.

Thus, now that you know that <u>boys need more attention</u> than girls, that doesn't mean that girls don't need to feel secure. Their more developed brains can pick up on problems, so it's important to make them feel secure as well, but maybe not in the same ways. Girls enjoy explanation and role play. When they play with dolls, they have a pretty good understanding of what bedtime means and why the doll should be put to bed and it works in a logical manner.

However, with boys, more affection is needed to reassure them that everything is alright. The undeveloped part of their brain doesn't understand as readily as the logical part of the female brain, so parents need to make allowance for this in that they would be expected to give more cuddles, more kisses, more attention to detail and perhaps a little more reassurance when it comes to bed time. If this is established at an early time in the child's life, it makes it much easier to impose strict bedtimes on boys at a later stage. The other thing to be aware of is that a mother may suffer from postpartum depression following having a boy as opposed to a girl. Again, one can only assume that there is a hormonal link somewhere, although reports are quite adamant that this is the case.

The structure of bedtime is something that is worth looking into. For example, it should not be a time when a toddler feels like he/she is being sent away. Instead of that, there are methods that you can use to help the child to get off to sleep. Reading a book together can be a bonding experience, as long as the child is aware of how much time you are going to give them at bedtime and is not encouraged to ask for more of everything. This can be the logical way for a child to extend bedtime, but if the rules are clear and a pattern is formed for the bedtime rituals, this helps the child to accept that bedtime is indeed a time when there is no room for negotiation but that this is also a time of sharing with the parents and they can be sure of love being shown toward them. Too many parents try to put children to bed and close the door, leaving the child wondering if he is loved or even scared of the dark because of the contrast between light and darkness and not being accustomed to it. Many fears in children are brought about simply because their imaginations conjure up all kinds of scenarios which can be dealt with by a different approach to bedtime.

Chapter Two: The Ideal Step by Step Bedroom Routine

As a toddler is learning, you need to introduce behaviors that he recognizes as being part of the going to bed process and a winding down of another day. Your toddler's body clock is not yet set and all of the steps I have outlined in this chapter will help you to help your toddler to establish those links. Later in the book I have mentioned about using charts to help your child to understand that certain things happen at certain times of the day, and that's not a bad idea. You can say that "Mr. Clock" says it's time to put the toys away, for example, so that the child does not feel that it's the parent's fault that play has come to an end for the day. Here is the ideal schedule for putting toddlers to bed in ideal circumstances. Bear in mind that you will have to make adjustments when you are traveling, when the child is not in his own home and at times of illness, but apart from that, the routine should become something the child becomes familiar with.

Step One – Toys get put away - This is a good habit. It clears up the play area and leaves the house tidy. In some homes, this may be on the ground floor and it's important what the house looks like. Invest in a huge toy box instead of expecting a child to sort through things and put them into certain cupboards as that may be a little difficult for the child to grasp. If you have drawing tools, these can all be placed into a plastic box so that they don't stain other things, but at the end of the day, all of the play things are to be put into the box. Mom can help with the clearing up because toddlers love to mimic adults and will be happier to join in rather than be expected to do all of the work themselves.

Step Two – Bath and Pajamas - This gets the child into the routine that he needs to be clean and relaxed at the end of the day. If you want to encourage your little ones to enjoy this time, invest in some floating toys and even bubble bath that is suitable for their delicate skin. This is a time when the child is preparing for what he knows lies ahead and parents should supervise the bathing process and wash the child's hair. It can be a fun time, but don't make it too rowdy as you are also getting ready to wind down for the day.

Step Three – Supper - It is known that kids who have supper sleep better. In the chapter relating to this you will see the kind of supper that is usual at this time of night. It is a light something just to stop hunger pangs and a drink but not too large. This is enough food for the night and will stop the child complaining about being hungry five minutes after being tucked in for the night. Supper should be a time spent sat down eating, rather than being active. If parents can sit down with the kids, this gives them the impression that they are not alone. After supper, make sure that one of you goes upstairs and draws the curtains to the nursery so that the bedroom ambiance is correct for sleeping. Check the bed and go back down to the children to encourage them to go to the bathroom and clean their teeth and have one last try at going to the toilet.

Step Four – Tooth Brushing and Toilet - It's a very good idea to make sure that your little one has a clean diaper for the night and this is the ideal time for that. Make sure that your toddler is encouraged to clean his teeth properly and to ready himself for bed. You may find that the child likes a little bit of independence, so I encourage parents to have a stool that the child can stand on. The more grown up a child feels at this age, the more the child feels in control of learning things like potty training and hygiene, so encourage your child to enjoy this part of the evening.

Step Five: Choosing your reading material together – You want to avoid any hurry at this stage. Take your time with your child and choose suitable reading material before placing the child into bed and tucking him in. The story should never be something that is going to wake him/her up, but should be read in a low voice, so that the child can hear, but also so that he relaxes while the words are read to him. He may enjoy looking at the pictures, but at bedtime, make this kind of interaction minimal because you don't want to wake him up. You can promise him that you can look through the book tomorrow at play time but make sure that you keep the promise as he/she will remember that you made it.

Step Six: Getting the room ready for the night – The room light should already be subdued, so when the reading is finished, tuck teddy into bed with your little one and ask him/her to look after teddy because teddy needs lots of love. Never skimp on a cuddle before you place the child into bed, because after the reading, all that is left is a little bit of affection and a kiss goodnight. The child knows that you are going to leave the room and this may prove to be a difficult time with boys. If it is, an extra cuddle won't go amiss, but the child does have to understand that bedtime is bedtime and there is really no negotiation.

Step Seven: Dealing with crying - It is quite normal for a child to whimper before they go off to sleep. They are tired, probably a little grouchy and now you are leaving them on their own in their bedroom and that makes their little hearts a bit anxious. However, although you may be monitoring the sounds, be aware that this may die down very quickly if the child is left to it. There are systems that have been devised whereby you are told by experts to ignore crying. However, if the crying gets too forceful, the child can get extremely distressed and I would never recommend that to anyone. Go in and cuddle the child if you have to calm him, but remember that placing the child in his bed for sleep is very important. Any other reaction will encourage the child to keep on trying to win your favor when it comes to being moved into the grownups bed.

You need to remember that psychological damage can come from fear and that this battle is about fear not about wits. If your child is a little uncomfortable with the level of light, perhaps you can adjust the light a little so that he feels more comfortable. Sit on the chair beside the bed. Sing a lullaby if you want to and you will notice that the child will gradually go to sleep. It may take a little bit of training, but the idea is that you gradually move yourself away from the side of the bed. You are still there to reassure but the distance between you should become more, so that you are able to leave the room and carry on with your evening without too much problem.

Safety considerations in the bed area – Make sure that the bed is not crowded in with toys and that there is nothing that can harm the child within the area of the bed. This should be a cozy place where the child can relax without turning over and hurting himself on sharp toys. You will know from the level of dribbles whether the child is teething and this may give you a clue about the discomfort of the child. If you pop in before you go to bed and notice that the pillow case is particularly wet, you can change it so that the wetness does not disturb your little one while he sleeps.

The reason that you leave changing the diapers until the last moment is so that the child has a chance to get through the night without the diaper becoming uncomfortable or wet or soiled. This helps the child to get off to sleep without the diversion of bodily needs. Most toddlers will respond well to a dry bed and are less likely to be woken by discomfort if the bed is dry and the diaper is clean.

Catering for the bodily needs of a toddler.

On average a toddler needs a total of 11 to 12 hours of sleep in a 24 hour period. Keep a diary note of the times that the child slept in the day and you will get a much better idea of how to adjust the daytime schedule to encourage more tiredness at night. This will change as the child grows, but for the time being it's important that you respect that need and that during the hours of being awake, the child eats food that is nutritious and gets plenty of outdoor exercise. This helps the child to get the most of healthy nutrition and fresh air and all of this contributes to how well the toddler sleeps. A happy child who has a well-balanced life will be easier to train than one who is not given sufficient exercise and has excess energy to burn when it comes to bedtime. That excess energy could be the reason for lack of sleep, so adjust the daytime schedule accordingly.

Remember, there is no bargaining when it comes to bedtime. Many parents do barter with their children by saying "Okay one more story" or "Okay you can come downstairs for another half hour" or by letting the child dictate the rules for bedtime. It has been proven time and time again that this isn't the end to the problem, but is the beginning. A child who knows that a parent

17

will bargain will be even more angry and upset when the parent decides that bargaining is not possible on certain nights of the week. Thus, you need to instill that just as a child eats his breakfast, he also needs to learn that certain actions are not negotiable. The ideal steps in this chapter are ones that will get you off to a good start. Involve the toddler in every single step including putting the toys away, sitting very still and quietly for his/her supper, going through the hygiene things like cleaning the teeth and going to the toilet and the child will have a better understanding of what is to be expected at bedtime.

The things that will sidetrack you are:

- Illness and how to deal with it
- Crying that seems irrational
- Signs that something is wrong and getting to the bottom of it
- Insecurity shown by the child in the way he/she acts out

Most of these are common sense things to deal with. For example, if you suspect illness then a visit to the doctor can reassure you. Crying that seems irrational can be dealt with by sitting by the child's bed and trying to work out what it is that is upsetting the child, without taking the child out of the bedroom environment. Sometimes, the child just needs to settle down with teddy and have the reassurance that mom or dad is there listening to them. You can also go through the different areas of the room to reassure the child that there is nothing to be afraid of. Introducing a lamp is a good idea for children whose fear seems to stem from being in the darkness, but be aware of where you place it so that it does not cast frightening shadows on the child's bed.

You will get to know this small child very well. You will know when the crying is just the whimpering of a child who doesn't want to go to bed and who is already tired and grumpy. You will also go through the stages of learning about teething and teething associated problems, but expect to have some sleep disturbance during the toddler stage as the child is going through changes. You also need to make sure that the bed is a safe environment for the child who has learned to get up and move off the bed during the night.

As a finale for this chapter, I want to show you a video of what toddlers can get up to at night if you allow them to. Having a two way communications system is a good idea coupled with a video camera, so that you are able to tell the child to get back to bed when things like this happen. This particular video always amuses me and I have experienced children who are every bit as adventurous at night time. What you need to make sure of is that the kids are safe and as long as you are happy that they are, the rest is merely childhood development and curiosity!

Chapter Three: Understanding why Parents Need Sleep

It may be obvious to some that a good night's sleep will give you the energy you need to get through the next day. However, in this day and age, many people stay up late anyway and take their phones or tablets to bed with them, keeping them up until all hours on social media or simply catching up with work. You need to understand it isn't just your toddler who needs sleep. You do and the quality of your sleep will, to a large extent, dictate what kind of attitude you have toward your kids in the morning. The fact that you have children at home who need your supervision puts you under even more strain than you would have experienced as a single person. You need to recover from the pregnancy and you also need to get beyond the changes that have happened in your life and these are not natural things for you to take onboard. Thus, sleep is more important now than it ever was before.

If you are not sleeping well, then you need to make sure that you set a time for going to bed and try to make the most of the peace and quiet of the evening to help to calm you. One way you can do this is to avoid watching loud television late at night or programs that are action-packed. Watch these when you are more awake and when you know you don't have to get up early in the morning. In a similar way, you may find that eating and drinking too late at night can make you lose sleep because your digestive system is still working while you are trying to relax. You need to do the best that you can to maximize the sleep that you are able to get because lack of sleep can make you:

- Irritable
- Irrational
- Increase your blood pressure
- Worry about heart health
- Forgetful

I know that the major subject of this book is toddler sleep but if you are not at your best, then you are not able to give the child the kind of support that he/she needs during the daytime and this may aggravate getting the toddler off to bed in the first place. Thus, you need to see that balanced sleep is important so that you are strong during the day and able to cope with all of the ups and downs of parenthood.

If you do find that you are having problems with sleep, it's a good idea to look at your lifestyle to find out where you may be going wrong. Stress is a huge factor and if you are stressed, it may be a good idea to seek help. That doesn't necessarily mean asking your doctor for medications. It means taking some me time to do things that help you to relax, such as yoga classes, go to the gym, go swimming or do things that help your body to find its rhythm. Yoga is useful because it teaches you a lot of the skills that you need to be a patient parent and it also helps you to feel stronger when faced with difficult situations. The gym can help, if your lack of sleep is because you are not getting enough physical exercise in your life. When you are at home looking after toddlers, sometimes you fall into bad habits and that's to be expected, but you can counter this by being aware of the lifestyle that you are living and making sure that you incorporate the following:

- Enough exercise

- Enough of the right kinds of foods
- Enough sleep
- Enough "me" time

If you do have a partner who is willing to take part of the load for part of the time, that's a good sign that you can get beyond these problems. If you are a single parent, then maybe it's time to enlist the help of family members so that you can get away from the things that are stopping you from sleeping and establish a good lifestyle routine.

Your toddler, at the end of the day, will benefit from your absence because you will be more even tempered, you will be more relaxed and you will feel more whole and refreshed. That's important because facing a bad tempered parent day after day can actually add to the problems rather than decreasing them.

Just as you have to prepare the toddler's room for him/her to sleep, you should also be aware of the need to make your room a haven in which you can get the sleep that you need. Make sure that your sheets are fresh, that the room is aired regularly and that the bedroom area is only used for sleep. It should be a relaxing place where you can wind down and rest when you need to and that's very important for a parent to do. Even if this means taking naps during the day, to help you when you have had bad nights, that's acceptable.

However, the overall aim is for you to sleep the required 8 hours per night without being interrupted by the toddler and without having to constantly get up to deal with what's going on outside of your room. In the next chapter, we will deal with getting the baby's room ready for the child to be comfortable at night. This is an important part of parenthood and the bond between mom and dad and the toddler. It's important to bear in mind that the needs of one child may not be the same as they were for another child. Thus we have covered this from all aspects. If your planning is done correctly and you bear in mind your own need for a good night's sleep as well as that of the toddler, chances are you can come through this period of their growing up unscathed. However, don't think you can do that if you deprive yourself of the sleep that you need. You need to be strong and healthy to deal with kids of this age, so look after you because in doing so, you are ensuring that they are looked after properly and they can't be if you are always every bit as cranky as they are.

Chapter Four: Getting the Toddler's Room Ready for Sleep

It's very hard for you to sleep when you are surrounded by clutter. When it comes to near bedtime, create a routine where the child is encouraged to help you to put everything away for the night. A huge toy box is a good idea. A neat bedroom that doesn't have a lot of junk all over the place will create a more relaxed atmosphere for the child and will help to tempt him/her to go to sleep instead of having their attention drawn to those things surrounding them.

Light

If you talk to your toddler, you can establish whether the toddler likes a little bit of light in the room. It's helpful from two viewpoints. One, it will stop the child from being afraid of the dark as a dim light can help to illuminate the room a little so that they are not afraid. The other viewpoint is that it doesn't give the child the excuse to have the door open, which is sometimes a mistake. When the child hears that people are still enjoying themselves without them being involved, often this causes the child to cry out for extra attention.

The bed

Some toddlers will have problems with wetting the bed. This is quite normal and can be dealt with during potty training.

However, for the time being, make sure that the cot has clean sheets and that there is nothing to distract baby while he is lying in the cot. It's a good idea to have a soft toy that the child can cuddle, though try to avoid anything that is too big which may scare the child or become a problem insofar as suffocation is concerned. The bed should be placed in an area where there are no drafts and where the child has no real distractions. You need to place a seat next to the cot, so that you can sit there and tell your child their evening story. Some people actually enjoy playing a little bit of music to the child when he/she is put to bed, so this chair will serve that purpose too.

When your child is either at baby or toddler stage, the most important thing that you can do is teach the child to put himself to sleep. That may sound a little strange, but they need to learn the body clock cycle as this is something that is new to them. Thus, their room or the place where they sleep has to become a part of the ritual of everyday life. That means that you need to be able to block out light, so they can distinguish between night and day. This also helps to cut down on distractions. Even if your baby goes to bed for an afternoon nap, you have to be able to blacken the room a little so that the light is softer and there is less distraction for the child.

There are several ways in which a baby learns to sleep on his own. You may find that your child has a natural tendency to suck his thumb, or may need that security blanket or special toy with him/her when going to bed, but that's okay. You may also find that rocking helps, but inevitably, you need to look at the things that the baby finds for himself as working toward good sleep.

In the nursery, the child should not feel cut off from everyone. You will need to make sure that you are there to reassure the child as they make their way through the processes that happen before sleep. However, if you make your routine one that the child can trust, the child is much more likely to respond in the way that you want him/her to respond, i.e. by sleeping.

You need to have spare sheets in the room and to make sure that just before bedtime, his/her nappy is changed so that there is no discomfort present to keep the child awake. If bedwetting occurs, don't make a big deal of it. Simply place the child into a safe position while you change the sheets and talk in tones that are reassuring. Never be mad at a toddler for wetting the bed. They have not yet learned to control that kind of thing and it takes time before this will happen. Simply change the bed and make sure that the bed smells fresh before placing baby back into the cot. I found the best way of preparing the nursery was to think of all of the bad things that can happen in the night and have all of the props needed within the room. If you find that you have to leave the nursery to get things, the chances are that the child will wake up as you wander from room to room with the child in your arms. Thus, if you can stay in the dim light of the nursery at all times and access the things you are likely to need, you have a much better chance of getting baby back to sleep again quickly and without too much trouble.

Be prepared with clean nappies, a changing mat, clean sheets, a clean dummy and everything you believe you will need during the night. Having these within easy reach is also important. Your child will eventually learn to sleep, but all of the effort that you put into the preparation is of paramount importance. If you also want to have an intercom system in the room, make sure that this is placed where you will hear if the baby has problems during the time that he/she is alone in the room. Remember that small whimpers are not a good reason to disturb the baby but by the same token, you do need to be aware if the child is ill or if there is something you need to do as a parent. Be aware of new things happening, such as teething problems or the problems that come after you change from bottle feeding your child to feeding the child solids.

If you have twins in the same room, try to avoid having the cots side by side. They will be aware that the other child is in the cot next to them, but discouraging playing together at night is a good idea. When the cots are side by side, one child will keep the other awake, so lining up the cots against the wall isn't such a bad idea. Remember too that with twins there is twice the potential for accidents as they may encourage each other out of their cots and thus there should be no excess cushions, encouraging this kind of activity.

Chapter Five: Sleep Basics

The amount of sleep your child gets makes a difference to his/her temperament the next day, so it's important to realize that sleep is needed and that it can be achieved even if it takes you some time to get the routine established.

The basics of putting babies or toddlers to bed are simple. They need to know that it's time for the end of the day routine. With toddlers, that means teaching them to clean their teeth and perhaps even going to the toilet before bedtime. The more independent you make your kids, the more they seem to respond well to changes. For example, why not invest in a small stool so that toddlers can reach their own toothbrush. Don't be critical. Be consistent and let them know what the routine involves. The nearer you can come to the same routine daily, the better.

Place the toddler into his cot, and then encourage the toddler to tell you what story they would like to hear. Perhaps you can even choose a book every night on the way to the cot. That way, they know you are not simply going to turn off the light and leave. Take time reading the story to the child. In dimmed light, this will probably send them off to sleep anyway, but if your child is extra active, that time spent reading will help to slow him down and give him the relaxation that he needs in order to get to sleep.

Cuddles before you place the child into the cot are an essential for both boys and girls. Making sure that the bed is comfortable and leaning forward to give your child a kiss goodnight, don't be tempted to join in more play at this time. That's why reading is chosen as the ideal night time routine – because it's quiet and it encourages them to relax. When you put the book down, lean over and kiss your child, and gradually start to leave the room. You may find that the child is quite happy in their bed, although with boys, often after a short time they start to cry or whimper. A small crying session is okay, but if the child is obviously more seriously affected than that, simply come into the room and don't talk. Simply be there. Stroke the child's head if you feel that the child needs a little reassurance, or tuck him back in if he has thrown off the bedclothes. He has to know that this is the time to sleep, so picking him up isn't an option at this time. If you do that, the child is learning something very valuable. He is learning that he can get his way by crying and that you will respond by giving him more hugs and perhaps even letting him stay up a little longer.

The less contact you have at this stage, the better. The child knows that you are there and you need to talk in a lulled voice so as not to wake him up fully. Whisper if you need to reassure him, but try to keep the child in the cot while you tidy around him, letting him know you are not far away. Little by little the child will learn that you are serious about bedtime and will resist less. The problem that some parents have is that the slightest whimper will get them picking the baby up and this really does disturb the sleep routine. Try to avoid that if at all possible.

What position should a child sleep in?

The child should be laid on his back with a very flat nursery pillow if any pillow is used. The reason that fluffy pillows is not a good idea is that they can stifle the child's breathing. If the child is at an age when he is able to roll over, that's okay, but always place the child on his back to sleep. There are some people who worry about the child vomiting and choking, but pediatricians are quite adamant that this is the best position for a child to sleep because a child will turn his head if he vomits and is less likely to choke than you think. However, cot death syndrome usually happens when children are placed on their sides or even face down on the mattress, restricting their breath.

This sleeping position is known as the "supine" position. It is important that the toddler or baby's feet are at the very bottom of the crib and that the sheets are tucked in tightly so that the child cannot wriggle and try to get further underneath the blankets. This prevents SIDs and is very important. However, as your toddler grows up a little, you will find that he will turn on his side regularly and as long as the blankets are tucked into the bottom of bed so that he cannot pull them over his face and the right kind of pillow is used, this should not cause a problem.

The use of a dummy

There are parents who use this to try to comfort a growing toddler or use it during the teething stages. It's not a good idea to use a dummy on a child over the age of 12 months, as this is when the child's teeth will start to form. If you really think that a dummy is helping the child to go to sleep, don't be tempted to use sugary substances on the dummy as this can be harmful to health. You also need to be aware of the cleanliness of the dummy and only use it for the purpose of going to sleep, rather than introducing it during the day simply to keep the child quiet. This is a period when the child is growing his teeth and sugar is to be discouraged at this stage as it can rot the teeth even before they are fully developed.

Clothing for bed

The child's clothing should be comfortable for going to bed. It is better to use cotton clothing that will absorb sweat rather than using anything containing wool which will not only encourage sweat but will also become too warm during the night. The garment worn should be comfortable. Try to avoid all in ones that are a little on the small size as these can make the child uncomfortable. For a baby, a cotton nighty is going to be the best because you have access to change the nappy easier but for toddlers, the all in ones are perfect because they keep the diaper in place even when the child wriggles. Make sure that the diaper is clean and dry at bedtime.

Chapter Six: Food to Eat Before Bedtime

Although we have mentioned that adults should not eat close to bedtime, you have to remember that small babies and toddlers are growing entities. They have an abundance of energy and the kind of food that you feed to your child will have an effect on the kind of sleep that the child gets. One of the desired hormones within the body that helps to induce a state of wellbeing is serotonin and there are certain foods that you can feed your toddler that contain this, a short time before the tooth brushing occurs. Yoghurts that are natural and without any coloring are ideal as these encourage the release of serotonin as does milk or a mild cheese, although do avoid the processed kinds of cheese that may have other ingredients that are not natural in them. Some of the toddlers that I have dealt with over the years loved a warm glass of milk, but don't overdo quantities since this may contribute to needing to pee in the night. Yogurt is far less likely to cause this problem but will help the digestive system while the toddler sleeps and the small pots particularly aimed at little people are ideal.

Try to avoid anything that encourages a sugar spike as this will give the child extra energy at a time when you would really rather the energy levels were lower. A rusk for example or a slice of toast are preferable to sweets of any kind. If you do serve toast, then make this taste a little nicer with natural honey rather than using jam. Dry crackers are also a great choice, though limit the amount of supper that is encouraged. In a way you are feeding the body's needs but you are also making sure that the child doesn't wake up too early demanding food. This only applies to toddlers, since babies are a totally different ballgame. However, you will have already established a routine as far as baby milk is concerned and this has the same effect.

If you choose to give your toddler fruit for supper, then try to avoid those fruits that are high in sugar content the plumb for those that release magnesium and also potassium as these will help the child to go through the night without cramps or discomfort. Bananas are also a good choice in small quantities as these contain tryptophan which helps in the release of serotonin. Food should not be given directly before bedtime, though there should be a period in the early evening when the child should be sat down for supper just after having put away all of his toys for the night and before being encouraged to clean his/her teeth. The quantities that you give the child should be small. These are only snacks and encouraging a child to eat too much at bedtime is not a good idea. Avoid cereals at all costs because many of these have sugar coating, which is far too likely to spike their sugar levels, and bedtime is not the right time to do this. Avoid white bread as well for the same reason. The more you encourage your little ones to eat the right kinds of foods, the better, but you need to know that example is paramount. If you want them to eat and enjoy healthy foods, make sure that you show the toddler that these are foods that are yummy to you too. Rather than giving a child a whole banana and then cutting it into smaller pieces and taking some away, prepare their supper on a plate with only the food that they are allowed to eat placed on it. This can stop any arguments from developing just before bedtime when the child is already grumpy. Teach your child to take his time with eating as indigestion can be a real problem if a child is encouraged to eat while walking around or eating too fast. Thus, supper should be a calm time that you spend together with your kids in the calm of the kitchen, away from temptation such as the TV.

Chapter Seven: Understanding Toddler Psychology

Toddlers don't like to feel that they are missing something. If you place a toddler into his cot and then have the door open, chances are that he can hear people downstairs still awake and having fun. It's obvious that the child is going to feel left out if you place him/her into this situation. Therefore, you need to know how the mind of a toddler works leading up to bedtime and what they will be thinking about as you go through the routine of supper, cleaning teeth and preparing for bed.

Children are not actually playing up when they start to protest at bedtime. There are all kinds of stories that have been devised to make parents believe that it's a battle of wits between the child and the grownups, but what they do not realize is that the bedroom is not yet a comfortable environment for the toddler who actually feels abandoned in the darkness and may actually be afraid of being alone. When you talk to people outside of the western world, they cannot believe how we treat our toddlers as it is quite normal in societies such as theirs to take the kid to bed in the same room as other people and these are folks who hardly ever have problems such as toddler tantrums, but there are ways that you can minimize these tantrums and help make your child feel safe in the environment of his/her bedroom.

If you race into the room every time the child makes a noise, he sees this as having achieved the required action and it's not a good idea to do that. However, it's also quite hard to ignore a child who is in distress. The way to get over this is to make sure that the environment the child is in feels safe to him. It's a big boy or big girl thing to have your own room and letting the child participate in putting the room together is a very good idea. There should be safe places for things. The toys obviously go in their box for the night, but your child needs to cuddle something and even if you believe your child to be a little old for cuddling, don't force the child to give up his soft toy too early. It's his protection for the night when the light goes out and is important to him.

Another way you can help the child to feel that he is not alone is to talk to teddy at the same time as putting the child to bed. Tuck in the child and tuck in teddy and the child feels that he has the company of a friend. I think that talking to the soft toys is very effective for addressing bad behavior in toddlers too. One particular child that I looked after was greedy about his toys. I showed him how sad teddy was about losing the use of these toys but did it in a very different way than you may expect. Teddy picked up all of the toys and placed them in his side of the play area and every time the toddler went to get something, teddy would show he was angry. Gradually, he learned that it's not a good feeling to keep things to yourself. Teddy can be a really good tool in dealing with psychological problems with a child and at bedtime, this is particularly relevant.

Another psychological thing with toddlers is that they like to feel that they are like grown-ups and will often copy parents. This is a useful tool to use at bedtime. Sit down and have supper with your children, and get them to clean their teeth without interrupting too much. In fact, if you do it with them, they learn from your example. A nice bath in the evening before bedtime will help to relax them before they go to bed, but more than anything else, they will start to get anxious toward bedtime because they know that they are going to be placed in a separate space from other people and this will play on their minds.

It's helpful if you have toddlers of similar age who can sleep in the same room as the children no longer feel that they are alone. However, avoid putting brothers and sisters into the same room if they are not of similar age groups, as this may impede the older child from having space needed to do things like homework or simply be on their own.

To a toddler, it isn't a natural thing to be parted from the people they trust and love. Thus, the bedtime routine gets to be a very hard thing for parents to have to deal with. Remember that this is a little person who is looking for reassurance and who just needs to feel comfortable in the space that he or she is in. I have dealt with children from all walks of life and one of the best tools that a parent can employ when it comes to settling a toddler into his own bed is to be reassuring and to be empathetic to the little person who finds it very strange to be on his/her own. Give reassurance. Tuck teddy in as well and make sure that the child is comfortable. After that, if you do need to look in from time to time, do so to reassure the child that you have not forgotten him/her.

You have to think of things in a very simple manner instead of trying to see the child as being intelligent enough to be taking you on in a battle of wits. If you lose your temper, that frightens the child, but not in a good way. You then expect the frightened child to sleep in a room with no one else there and that's not at all logical and can cause the child psychological damage. However, if the child feels safe and loved and has teddy to go to sleep with he will feel safer and will not be as troublesome as a child who is told off for making a noise.

If you make the routine of bedtime a fun thing instead of a dread, you will have far less problems with your toddler and you will be able to look for teddy together and tell your bedtime stories, knowing that your toddler knows teddy is his friend and that he is never really being left alone in the darkness at all. Even leaving the door a crack open may help but you can only tell this by judging your child's reaction to the first couple of nights of being alone.

Chapter Eight: Dealing with Siblings

In some small way, it can help you to get over the bedtime blues if you have kids whose age is not that distant from each other. A two year old and a three year old can sleep quite happily in the same room and the same routine should be used for both children. Bedtime should be at a marked time and there should be no favoritism shown toward one child over the other. Both children should be placed in their beds ready for their night time story. You may have some arguments about who chooses the story for the evening, but you can use logic for this and let the children take turns with choosing. Never appear to be more favorable toward one child, as both of these toddlers are important.

I said earlier that it wasn't a good idea to have kids of different ages in the same room although if you are stuck for alternatives it can work, but only if you plan for it correctly. It's not fair to ask an older child to share the room with a toddler if the older child needs a little bit of space for privacy and for doing homework and for having friends come to stay. Therefore, try to avoid having kids of different ages sharing if it is at all possible. One of the mistakes that parents make when it comes to bedtime is expecting the older child to take responsibility for the younger child and that's not fair. It's not the older child's responsibility to look after the younger child and although they may seem willing to do that, it's better if you can treat all of your kids equally. That means allowing the older child to have the space to do the things that older kids do.

The argument that can occur when you have two toddlers in the same room is that there can be arguments over toys. The best way to avoid this getting in the way of the bedtime routine is to make sure that play is confined to a different area from the bedroom and also that each child has his/her teddy that definitely belongs to them. You may have seen jokes about how kids need their security blankets, but it's not really a joke to the child. It's a serious need and if you find one of your kids does hold onto something for security, then you need to learn to deal with this at bedtime. As long as the toy or item does not cause any kind of danger in the sleeping area, then it's okay for the kids to have their security with them over the course of the night.

One particular child that I looked after loved to take his mom's sweater to bed and I think that this made her feel closer to him. If there was any hint that this was going to be taken away to be washed, he would really object, so this had to be done in the daytime when he hadn't noticed that it was missing. It's important to make sure that siblings do not argue and the best way to do this at bedtime is to sit down and read to the siblings and make sure that both are equally involved in the storytelling process. Your voice should be relatively low in pitch so that it does not excite the children before they go to sleep. The story that you choose should also be one that does not give the child food for thought that may get their imaginations going wild just as they are going off to sleep.

Chapter Nine: Sleep Training A – Z

When your baby comes home from the hospital, the chances are that you will have the baby sleeping in the same room as you. It's practical and it's the best way to ensure that the baby is safe. It's also a good way to have access to the baby for feeding. If you can place the cot near the bed where you can reach out and get the baby for feeding sessions, this is the best way to do it because it minimizes the amount of interrupted sleep that you get. When the baby has been fed and is ready to sleep again, he can be placed back in the crib to go to sleep. Be aware of his need to be winded and also the need to rock the cradle until baby has gone back to sleep.

The majority of this book is about toddlers and they are quite a different story. You may have the toddler in your room for a while until you have prepared a room for them, but if this is the case, make sure that you involve the child in the preparation of his/her room so that they look forward to a time when they have their own space, rather than worrying about it. When a toddler is placed into bed, he/she needs to be tucked in. Then, you need to turn down the lights and read a story to the child. If the child gets out of the supine position, put him/her back into that position and continue with the story.

The routine that you use should be the same one as is used every night and if there are times when you are not going to be there to do that, it's a good idea to explain to a babysitter so that the babysitter can do what the child is accustomed to. The whole bedroom routine and training consist of the following elements:

- Getting ready for bed and putting toys away
- Bathing and putting on pajamas
- Cleaning the teeth and brushing the hair
- Going to the toilet/ or at least changing diapers
- Getting the room ready for the night and closing the drapes

The toddler needs to know what is going on and should trust it. If you change the routine too many times, the toddler can get disorientated and very irritable. Particularly boys find a change in routine difficult for their minds to cope with. Thus when you are training a toddler, from day one of the routine that surrounds their independent sleeping should take on the same format. Encourage the child to enjoy the room that is theirs. The one thing to remember is that the psychological factor does come into it. You cannot place a child in the bed and then leave and close the door. The child needs to be settled. Place the child into the bed, lying down and start your story telling. It's a good idea if both parents can take part but if this is not possible, the child should at least be given the opportunity to say goodnight to both parents.

After the story, the child should be encouraged to look after the teddy or the toy that the child has chosen as his friend. If you work on the basis that the bear is smaller than the child and needs all the love the little one can give him, the child will respond well and will be happy to be tucked in with the toy. This is an age when a child doesn't really understand much about relationships except for what he learns during his play time. You can use the teddy to give examples of good behavior and also make the bear into his trusted friend. That way, when bedtime comes, the toddler does not feel all alone in the world when the door is closed for the night.

It's a good idea to have the light ready for the night before the story telling, so that the child's eyes get accustomed to the dimmed light of the room. You can have a baby monitor in the room but don't make a big deal about it. Just check that it is switched on and that it is monitoring the baby. If you have already set the angle, you don't need to play around with it. When the story is finished and the bear is tucked in with the child, a kiss goodnight seals the deal for some kiddies, while others may cry for attention if this is the first time that they have been left on their own. There is a way to get the child used to the cot and you can do that during the daytime when it's nap time. Close the drapes and make the light dimmer but carry on doing housework around the child's room and adjoining area, so that he gets used to the fact that you are not far away. What this does is help the child to trust the cot environment.

If the child does cry and you feel that it is warranted to check on him/her, then open the door slightly so that you don't actually have to make a lot of noise going into the room. It's a mistake to turn the light on or to make a lot of noise as toddlers have oodles of energy and all you are doing if you change the ambiance of the room is wake up that energy. Talk to the child in a whisper and tuck the child in again. Listen to what he has to say. Don't be too quick to leave the room. You can sit by the cot for a while so that the child knows that you are there. Little by little, as the sleep gets deeper, you will be able to move out of the room and the chances are that the child will sleep for the rest of the night.

One thing that you should be aware of is that children do tend to wake when daylight happens. It's not that they have a built in clock yet, but once they have had a decent night's sleep, their energy levels are higher again and you may find that difficult at first, but you will get used to the rhythm of their day, little by little. You should establish with a child from baby age the difference between night and day and open the drapes to greet the day. It takes a while for a child to understand the sleep cycles that they need to go through. Their body clocks have not yet adjusted to life and by making a clear distinction between night and day, you are teaching them the way that life works and allowing them to find their own rhythm to life.

Chapter Ten: Sleepwalking and Nightmares

Did you know that as many as a third of all kids sleepwalk or have nightmares at some stage? It's true and although it can be a little scary, you do need to know how to behave when this happens and how to protect the child from any harm that they are likely to do to themselves while sleepwalking. Here are some safety measures that you can take to safeguard your child in the event of sleepwalking, but it's a good idea to have these in place anyway in case the toddler manages to get out of their cot and walk around before you are awake in the morning.

Place a gate against the top of the stairs

This should be a priority anyway. When toddlers try to get down the stairs, there are chances of an accident. Thus, having a gate means that they can't get any further than that gate and are less likely to have problems. One thing you should be aware of is that older toddlers may be tempted to try to get over that gate, so the further away from the top of the stairs you can place it the better. It is far better to make sure that the gate is very secure at all times and that the toddler is aware of why it is there. You can't stop a child from trying to take chances, but you can make the place relatively safe. Another area you should look at is hurdles that they may trip over if they sleepwalk. Of course, this means keeping the house a bit tidier but that's a good thing and makes your housework easier anyway, so it's a commonsense measure to take.

Be aware that when a child is sleepwalking, his/her eyes may be open but they may not be aware of walking. Thus, be careful not to wake the child as this may frighten the child. One of the main reasons for sleepwalking is fitful sleep or a sleep routine that is not working for the child. In the case of this being the case, perhaps you need to think about getting the child to bed earlier or making sure that the child has less napping time during the day, so that they are relatively tired at night. Physical exercise during the day and fresh air also helps a child to become worn out enough to sleep. Thus, make sure that your child does have regular outdoor exercise, even if this is just a walk to the park.

The Royal Children's Hospital has some great advice for parents and this is to avoid waking the child and to do the following when the child is sleepwalking:

- Redirect the child without making any movements that may wake the child.
- Make sure that the sleep routine is adjusted to suit the child.
- Lock windows and doors to stop any danger areas from being available to the child.
- Do not let a toddler who sleepwalks sleep in a bunk bed, particularly in the top bed.

There is some anti-social behavior that can be involved in sleepwalking. The child may urinate, although with a toddler, if you make sure that the diaper is clean and secure before the child goes to bed, this limits the possibility. However, when you place the child back into his bed, you should make sure that the sheets are dry and that the diaper is clean so that the child benefits from going back to sleep relatively unscathed by the sleepwalking.

One of the worst things that you can do if your child has a temperature is to encourage the child into your bed. Many children who sleepwalk have nightmares because of the high temperatures that they reach during the night and the added temperature of your bed may worsen the situation. In the case of a child having nightmares, be reassuring and make sure that teddy is there to help make the child feel safe once he/she is safely back in bed. You may find that the child has been frightened by shadows and you can adjust the lighting a little bit and even make a game of looking everywhere to reassure the child that there are no baddies in their bedroom and that everything is safe. You may also find that the child will benefit from a glass of warm milk, but not too much. Have a small drinking cup with a spout available so that you can provide the child with this comforting drink without having it spilt all over the bed sheets. There's nothing worse than the stale smell of milk.

When to get a doctor involved

This isn't always necessary but if you find that your toddler is having episodes regularly or more than twice a week, there may be an underlying problem that a doctor can help you to discover. Similarly, if you find that the toddler is actually urinating in unusual places, talking this through with a doctor can help you to decide on necessary action, although your response to this happening should never be one of anger or frustration as this can further the problems that are already existing. Remember bedwetting can happen at any age up to 10 years old, so don't be hard on your kiddie if this happens. Simply change the sheet and move on. The problem here is that if the toddler thinks you are going to shout at him when this happens, it may actually make the situation worse and scare the child.

The important thing to remember is that sleepwalking is a sign of something and you need to pick up on the reasons why it is happening. Do not try to wake the child and remember that the child will have very little recollection of sleepwalking in the morning. Thus making a fuss about it can actually induce more of the same kind of behavior because it may confuse the toddler. If you have more than one child sleeping in the same room and this happens, make sure that the floor area of the bedroom is always tidy so that the child does not hurt himself or fall over, thus waking the other child.

Chapter Eleven: Dealing with Medical Problems

There will be times during the childhood of your kids when you are concerned about health problems. For example, if a child catches a cold, it may be worrying for new parents who will be concerned about the child being able to breathe at night. In a case like this, there are creams that you can use safely on the toddler's chest that help them to breathe easier. If you feel that your child has a high temperature, it's also wise to dress the child suitably for his illness. There is nothing worse than sweating all night with a fever in bed-clothes that are too warm and that are uncomfortable. It's also a good idea to keep the bedroom aired and there's nothing worse for a toddler than to be left in a room that's stuffy when they feel so bad.

If the child is ill, chances are that he/she will want to sleep during the day and that's where problems can occur because it interrupts the need to sleep at night. You may find that your toddler suffers from the following symptoms but these are common symptoms from a cold and you should not be too concerned at first about them:

- Stuffy nose
- Dry cough
- Headache
- Mild fever
- Tiredness and bad temper

You have to place yourself in the shoes of the youngster. It's a miserable time and the child can feel really ill. A cold can typically last up to ten days and there are different ways to deal with toddlers of different ages.

Kids up to one year old

Since these are kids who need to sleep on their backs, and who cannot blow their noses, you may need to use a saline solution especially for the purpose of helping to loosen the mucus in the nose of the child. Ask your pediatrician about a suitable one for a child of that age. You may find that a suction bulb is a good investment because this helps you to suck out the mucus so that the baby can sleep more easily. If you do need to raise the pillow, don't be tempted to put another pillow into the actual bed on top of the mattress. It is a better idea to raise the bed head by placing a pillow under the mattress so that there is little chance of suffocation.

Kids from One Year to two years

These are your toddlers and they need extra attention when they are feeling the snuffles. It's a good idea to teach your toddler to blow his nose. You can do this by demonstrating how you do it on yourself as toddlers do love to copy what they see adults do. Raising the head is useful because this allows the child to breathe but if you are using a bed, then the kid can have an extra cushion, while if the toddler is still in a crib, then use the method that I described above where the mattress is raised by placing a pillow under it. Nasal spray will help to loosen up the mucus. However, if the child has a cough, try to use a cream on his chest so that he breathes this in during the course of his night.

It is important that you are extra loving to your child during the time that he/she has a cold, but the routine of your lives should not be too affected. Sure, look in on him/her more often if you are concerned, but it really is best to ensure that the child goes to bed at the same time and that he/she follows the same night time routine as normal. If you vary away from this, the child will work out that it can be to his/her advantage to be ill for longer and they may play on this extra attention. When you do visit the child in the night, don't take the child out of the bed if there is no need to do this, since this may wake the child up and make him less prone to go back to sleep.

Other Illnesses

It's a good idea to try and keep kids away from pharmaceuticals as much as possible, though some illnesses do call for them. Avoid using over the counter meds for your toddler since it's easy to give too much and they may not be as effective as those given by a doctor. If the doctor does prescribe drugs for your toddler, you need to keep these at a safe distance from the child who may mistake them for sweets. Respect the quantities prescribed and never overdo the drugs thinking that it will help baby to sleep.

When dealing with illness always take the advice of your pediatrician as he will know best what is suited to dealing with your child's own particular illness. This is particularly relevant to children who are suffering from illnesses that require hospital treatment. You should always respect the advice given by the experts, since they know how a child is likely to react to certain operations or as an after effect of having had a certain illness. Remember that childhood illnesses can get you down and it's a good idea not to vary your routine too much simply because of these. If you have a child at home all day, don't be tempted to prolong the daytime sleeping as this will interfere with their night time routine and you may find that the child becomes cranky and difficult to handle.

Chapter Twelve: Vacations and Away from Home Time

These are times when it can be very difficult to get a toddler off to sleep. If you are traveling in a car, then try to time the travel so that the toddler feels sleepy. This can mean traveling at night but it's a good idea to cater for the sleep, by having somewhere the child can stretch out comfortably and still adhere to the same kind of timetable that he/she has at home.

You can even go as far as stopping at a café to allow the child to clean teeth and to have a snack before bedtime just as he would at home, but make sure that the snacks are similar to those he is accustomed to. If these means carrying a little bit of fruit with you, that's not a bad idea and most people are very understanding about not giving a child a full meal in the evenings. The parents can eat and the child can simply have the snack that he associates with being near bedtime.

You have to appreciate that children in a new environment will be curious about what's happening around them. If you are able to lie the child down to sleep, bear in mind also that some children do suffer from travel sickness and make sure that you have squared this up with his doctor before you leave, so that you know what to do if the child suffers from motion sickness. Happily, most of the kids that I have dealt with in my life have actually enjoyed the motion of the car and have slept very well. The point of the whole exercise of travel is that it is timed in such a way that it causes minimum disruption to all of the timings you already have in place with the child. Traveling with a cranky toddler can be an absolute nightmare, so when you are booking flights or going long distances, try to work out a route that disrupts their routines as little as possible.

In flight, you may find that the child wants to look around and has the same level of curiosity as he would in any new environment. Try to get seats by the window so that you can show him the view and talk him through the different things that happen during the flight. If you are only flying a short distance, then the best time to travel is going to be in the afternoon. The reason for this is that the child is awake and although he may be a little cranky, he is still able to participate during the voyage and you can still use your same routine when you get to your destination, making sure that the child is in bed at the usual time and does not expect to be able to stay up late just because mommy and daddy are in a different place.

When staying with relatives, make sure that they know what your routine is. If you find that they eat later than you normally do, try to feed the toddler separately, so that his digestion is not upset by changes. Most people are quite understanding when it comes to feeding your child and will know that you know best.

There are several things that you will need at hand when you are traveling with a toddler and it's a good idea to pack these separately so that you have access to them at all times:

- Clean diapers
- A plastic bag to place used diapers in
- Creams and lotions used for care of the child's skin
- A bottle with a suitable drink for the child when needed

- Snacks that are healthy and that will not up his energy levels
- Changes of clothing in case of sickness

When you have the added responsibility of having a child, your whole life changes and that includes your vacation time. You will also find that relatives, although well meaning, will also disrupt the routine if you let them. It's a good idea to state what time the toddler goes to bed, the kind of TV that you do not encourage him watching and make sure that the child becomes familiar with the room in which he/she is going to sleep. In a situation like this, I think it isn't a bad idea to sleep the child in the same room as you because for a child, that new environment can be very scary. If you carry glow lights with you, these are small sockets that plug in and light up the room. They really do not take up much space and can help the child to feel less afraid of the strange environment into which he is placed.

The important things for the toddler are to know what the routine is and that this is unchanging. He will still be expected to bathe, clean teeth, eat supper and will still have that moment of reading with his mom or dad before being expected to go to sleep. Don't forget teddy. Remember he is a very important part of the child psychology of sleeping and will make the child feel safe and not alone. The first thing to pack when you go anywhere will be that teddy because it's your child's friend and that friend can come in very handy when you are trying to get your child to sleep in a new environment. A child will cling to the familiar, so make everything that happens as normal as possible.

If your child is going to stay with grandma and grandpa, then let them know the routine that you live by because often well-meaning grandparents who want to spend as much time as possible with their grandchildren will not know how important that routine is and may throw the whole routine out of the window if they don't know about it. It isn't an intentional ploy on their part. It's merely that they are not accustomed to the way that you do things. At the end of the day, if the child plays up while you are traveling, he will know that it doesn't matter where in the world he is. Bedtime is bedtime and there is no negotiation as far as this one element of his life is concerned. The story reading could help him to look forward to the next day of vacation, but don't over-excite the child and then expect him to be able to settle down. Remember, peace and calm are necessary even for adults to sleep so for a toddler it's even more important.

Chapter Thirteen: Why Some Toddlers Have a Hard Time Sleeping

You have to understand the psychology of a child but you also need to know that each child is very different and there may be underlying reasons why a child cannot sleep. Let's look at some of the common reasons as these may give you clues as to why your toddler finds it so hard to go to sleep.

Reliance on being with people – This is a common reason why toddlers suffer from anxiety. It's not natural for them to be separated from their parents. In other countries, toddlers don't have the same fear of sleep because they sleep with their parents or in a room with other family members. As society has evolved and toddlers in the western world now have their own rooms, unfortunately, their approach to this phenomenon has not changed with it. The child needs that bond of feeling within a safe distance of parents. Perhaps you can make the nursery in an adjoining room to your bedroom so that the child does not feel so isolated. However, you must understand that this is a real fear in the mind of the child. The insecurity of lying in a darkened room is hard for toddlers and they may even be afraid. Thus, you need to make the bedroom as toddler friendly as you can without creating too much drama like shadows that move or noise from outside the room that distracts the mind of the toddler.

What you may not be aware of is that sleep is a habit and that habits can be adopted, but if you want your toddler to adopt the habit of sleep, you have to gear life around it. Thus, calming down activity in the evenings helps. Having a routine helps and this can be helped by a chart where the child sees pictures of himself doing different things at different times. Drawing a clock and explaining everything step by step helps the child to see that it isn't a case of you neglecting the child, but that the clock dictates what happens at what time. His sleep needs to be a habit and until you break the ice and the child relents and makes it one, you have no chance at all to expect the child to simply adhere to instructions because you told them to.

The chart that you make can include all kinds of activities. For example, you can show the toddler the chart when it's time to get up and get dressed and show him the picture of the sun shining into the room telling him that it's daytime. Then you can add things like meal times and putty times but try to do this on a pin board so that you can add things to it as the child gets a little older and has more understanding of how it all works.

Deciding on a bedtime

The best bedtime for a child who is a toddler is between 6.30 and 7.00. The reason for this is that the child is not too tired to actually go to sleep. When a child is overtired, this makes the body produce adrenaline and that's the last thing you need because it energizes the child and may cause him to wake up after only a short while in the bed. Bedtime should always be associated with darkness, so the drapes need to be pulled. If the child likes a little light, then use a glow light to comfort him because these allow him to relax without making him pay too much attention to everything that is around him in his room. If your toddler naps during the day, then you may need to make his official bedtime a little later to ensure that the child does sleep though no later than 7.30 to 8.00 and try to wean off the daytime naps in favor of nighttime sleeping.

Introducing white noise

White noise is a noise that the child hears but is comforted by. It's not quite the same as the child hearing noises from outside the room and is a relaxing noise that will not wake baby when he goes through a patch of lighter sleep. The sleep cycle of a child goes through different phases and the white noise is simply a comforting sound in the background that encourages the mind of the child to continue to relax, rather than being woken by other sounds that have more of an invasive nature. You can get some great recordings of white sound and there are even some on YouTube if you want to use those. However, consistency is important so having a recording playing in the background of the nursery is a much better idea than combining it with pictures on a screen which will distract the child.

Keep your napping schedule in place

For children going through the toddler stage, naps are an important part of the day because children have spurts of energy following by hunger, followed by the need to nap. It's a good idea to have an established time for a child to nap. The fact that your child will not go to sleep means that the toddler is too cranky. He has gone over the edge of needing sleep and if you adjust your nap time to a period just after lunch, this is a good period for you to get a break and for your toddler to get used to the peaceful calm of sleep. Nap time can take place in his room or you can even encourage the child to nap in a place where you are present as this gives them the extra security that they need in order to learn the habit of sleeping. If they open their eyes and things around them are still normal, they are more likely to lull themselves back to sleep. That's why nap time is important. It's a learning curve for your child to learn the art of putting themselves to sleep. Lying on the pillow and relaxing in clothing that is comfortable also helps them to develop this habit, which can later be transferred to the bedroom area at bedtime. Naps teach the child to see sleep as something they want rather than something that is enforced. Thus, the importance for kids under the age of three cannot be underestimated. Don't be tempted to take away that nap time because when you do, you create a situation where the child is too tired to sleep at night and the body is sending him all the wrong signals and releasing adrenaline which will fire up his energy and make him even more cranky.

Teaching a child to sleep

This is quite important if you have a toddler who doesn't seem to get it that he needs sleep. The idea is to program the sleep and let the child know, when it's daylight it's time to get up and when it's night time, it's time that everyone goes to bed and gets to sleep. What may confuse the child is the noise of activity beyond his room, so you need to make the sleep process a gradual one where the toddler is leaning to relax and sleep on his own.

Sleep training for difficult toddlers

You can start to do this by placing the child onto the sofa beside you, all wrapped up and warm and ready to sleep. The child may need contact with you, so resting his head on your knee is perfectly acceptable. When you find that he sleeps in that manner, move him over to a position where a cushion takes the place of your lap. Then try a little distance. If you want to do this without causing the child concern, why not have something in your hands, so that there is less space for the child to place his head on your lap. You can place a cushion next to you and reach out and touch the child occasionally to give him the reassurance that he needs to get off to sleep. Little by little distance yourself from the toddler and encourage good sleep by making sure that the child knows this is sleep time and there should not be too much noise in the room. I once had one child who was really too stubborn to want to go to sleep and devised a way where we competed to see who could go to sleep first. The atmosphere of the room was calm, we each had a cushion and we both tried our best to go off to sleep. Because the insecure child knew that I was there with him, he was able to get off to sleep much quicker than I had thought he would be. Gradually impose separation. Gradually encourage the child to learn to nod themselves off to sleep and you have a very winning situation on your hands. A child who learns the process of sleeping is one who will not have too much trouble at night so nap time is a good time to practice sleeping and actually getting the mind into the right mindset to sleep.

Having something to look forward to

With toddlers who were difficult, I found that having a routine works very well. For example, if you know that your toddler wants to watch a favorite cartoon on the TV, make sure that this doesn't happen until after the routine of having a nap. It gives the child something to look forward to, but it also means that they learn early that the cartoon isn't going to happen until the nap is over and done with. While some may see this as bribery, it works very well because the child knows that when he wakes up, there will be something very worthwhile to wake up for and is more inclined not to fight the process of sleeping.

The toddler who cries at night

The jury is firmly out when it comes to what is the right way to deal with toddler crying at night. However, I can say from my own extensive experience that there are two things you have to bear in mind.

1) **If you leave the child to stew,** you are actually affirming their worst fears and the child does not get a chance to externalize these fears or rationalize his feelings. To my mind that's the worst response that you can give to a crying toddler. If you go into the room and ask the toddler what's wrong, you validate their feelings and you can go through their fears with them and prove to the child that they are unfounded, thus allowing those fears to come out and allow the child to relax.

2) **A hysterical child needs parental guidance.** Do not shout at the child as this makes the hysteria worse or can even worse set psychological problems into the mind of your little one. Calm the child. Talk to the child and do hold the child while they get over the hysteria. There are those who argue that this encourages a child to be hysterical at bedtime, but it doesn't really do that. What it does is show the child that you care and you can rationally go through what the child is feeling and put

things right in his mind. "I think there are monsters in my room." Go through the room with the child and make a point of showing him that there is no such thing. Imagine the child who believes there are monsters lying in the dark and listening to a parent shouting at him. The parent also becomes a monster and that makes the situation worse. Looking through all the places a monster can hide helps you to show the child that his thoughts are unfounded and calm him down. In a case such as this, it's even more important that you child has a friend to go to bed with him/her and this is where the favorite teddy comes in very handy indeed.

"Teddy has looked and there are no monsters."
"Teddy will look after you now, so don't worry. You have your friend with you."
"Cuddle teddy so he doesn't get scared by you crying."

You can really comfort a child without taking the child out of the room and back into your living room. If you do change the territory, it kind of gives the child the wrong message. The whole idea of night is sleep and if you can encourage that by addressing the child's fears, it's a much better way forward.

3) **You need to create calm**. If this means that you have to take the child out and rock the child in your arms, make sure that you have a comfortable chair from which you can reach the bed. Rocking gently takes time, but the more time you spend on this at this stage, the easier it becomes for the child to accept that sleep is necessary. When you notice that the child is beginning to sleep, place him back into his bed, and sit beside him for a little while until you are sure that the child is sleeping soundly. The Ferber method may work for some, although I consider there are better ways to do this by showing a toddler a lot of love and reassurance. It has always

worked for me and the children that I have helped through this stage moved on toward having a healthier attitude toward sleep than those children that were actually shut away and ignored.

4) **Never give in to unacceptable behavior** – A child who has had supper and who has had a drink is less likely to scream for food or drink at night. Thus, the whole routine of bedtime should revolve around getting the child ready for bed and sleep, rather than setting yourself up for potential problems. It's a good idea to keep food separate from the bedroom so that the child knows this isn't a place to eat. If your child has had supper and a drink and is still showing signs of thirst or hunger, the only things that you should give the child are a drink of water or a dry rusk, so that the child does not get the idea that bedtime is a time to scream for extra attention.

Many parents make the mistake of giving in, believing that they are being kind but they are actually teaching the child bad habits and not allowing the child to learn the art of rocking himself to sleep. For younger kids, a rocking crib is a great investment because they tend to be lulled by the motion of the crib and tend to go off to sleep easily. However, when your kid transfers from this to a larger bed, you need to teach him alternative methods of rocking so he can still achieve the same thing. One is cuddling his teddy and rocking the teddy to sleep. One is by making sure that the child is very comfortable and talking in a low whispering voice about things that fill the child's dreams with nice thoughts. Storytelling helps to do this, but be careful that the books that you choose for bedtime wind down naturally and the child will almost certainly be asleep by the time that you turn the last page of the book.

If your toddler is one of those who has a hard time sleeping, there will always be a reason. Don't ignore it, but try to address is. For example, the child who is teething may find it difficult to sleep because his gums hurt. Thus usually happens to younger kids and you should never deal with teething by giving the child something that is sweet to suck on. A lot of parents use a dummy dipped in honey but I would advise against this at bedtime, as this brings the sugar in the blood up to a certain level, which is not conducive with sleep. It is far better to use a pacifier during this period, but use it naturally or with a product given to you by your pediatrician.

It's worthwhile also to have the child checked for problems with their ears as it may not be teething that is keeping the little one awake. In a case such as ear problems, the pediatrician will be able to help you and reassure you of what is causing the lack of sleep and what can be done to encourage good sleeping habits. Remember, each toddler has their own problems and you, as a parent, need to be very aware of what those problems are so that you can address them and allow the child to have the peace of mind he needs to get off to sleep at night. Do not be tempted to give children any over the counter medications as you may not have your diagnosis correct whereas one appointment with your family doctor can sort out what's going on with your little one and get the child back to his sleep routine in a quicker and more effective manner.

Sleep Apnea or breathing problems

Toddlers may be afraid to go to sleep because of having breathing problems and if you can monitor this, it's a very good idea. The things to look out for are loud snoring or spurts of breath, where the child seems to have problems breathing. Breathing can affect the child's learning, growth and sleep so it's important to address any issues that you feel your child has with breathing straight away. Sleep apnea is something that toddlers usually grow out of very rapidly so it's not something to worry about. However, it's a good idea to talk to your doctor about it in case further investigation is needed to measure the extent.

Other potential breathing problems

Many kids suffer from asthma in this day and age and you may find that you are concerned about your child's breathing. It is likely that you will pick up on this during the day as well as at night, but it's something that needs to be addressed as quickly as possible in order to make sleeping easier for the child and to take away a lot of the stress that comes with this terrible malady. The first tool that you need to have in the home is a thermometer so that you can test your child's temperature and note when the child exhibits a high temperature.

If your child has a fever or has breathing problems for more than a couple of days, then do seek out advice from your doctor who will be able to eliminate certain potential illnesses from your list of worries. You may need to make adjustments to allow for asthma, such as limiting the child's contact with allergens that encourage the breathing problems, but these are fairly easy to overcome. Your doctor will be able to tell you if this is a real problem. Did you know that kids who are brought up with animals are actually less likely to suffer from asthma in the first place? Their bodies become more tolerant and it's not a bad idea to introduce pets, but before you do, have your child checked for breathing difficulties so that you can eliminate asthma as a potential cause. I did not include this in the illness area of the book, because it's not a sleep induced problem, but it can be a problem that parents do need to be aware of when it comes to a child having tantrums at bedtime and having difficulty with coughing and wheezing.

You are always better inquiring why a child cannot sleep by observing what happens with the child and whether the problems being encountered are psychological, physical or simply lack of routine. When you work out which it is, you will be able to address the problems and get your little one back on track and ready to learn the sleep process.

Chapter Fourteen: Problem Solving and Taking Care of Mom and Dad

You may think that the focus of this book is the toddler, but you'd be wrong. I have seen many marriages become less successful because all of the attention is given toward the toddler and the parents have actually put themselves out of the picture. The parent's needs are as important because a tired parent will not be a very patient one. The strength of the relationship also makes the family for the toddler a lot more secure so if both parties are happy, then the toddler will be happier too. However, how do you balance out parent responsibilities with actually allowing yourself the person freedom that you both need?

The home - You do need to strike a happy balance here and if you and your partner can get together to work out duties that can be done on an everyday basis, this really helps. There will be cleaning to be done and the neater you can kccp your home, the easier all of these tasks become. If you and your partner can learn to put things away after you have finished with them, this helps to make the home safer for the toddler too. It's good fun to do things like this together. Invest in a dishwasher as it's a major argument that should be doing the dishes. This makes it easier to get menial tasks out of the way. You also need to invest in a good laundry room with plenty of hanging space, so that laundry becomes easier. The child's clothing will cause you a lot of extra washing and you and your partner can take it in turns to wash and hang out the clothes, both taking responsibility for things that are not that much fun to do.

The other thing that you need to decide is how to split money and spare time. I know you will think it a joke when I mention spare time, but with many people telecommuting, working from home is a real possibility, which puts more money in your pockets to actually enjoy yourselves more. Having a child is not the end of the social life as you knew it and you need to be able to relinquish responsibility sometimes and make sure that you have plenty of "us" time. Go on a weekly date or visit friends without the toddler in tow because it's important that the main caregiver of the child has time with adults. It can become very dull indeed when the only person there is to talk to is a toddler!

As your children get older, you need to strike some kind of deal with your partner that you are both on the same page as far as any kind of parenthood goes. If a toddler gets the impression that he can get something out of dad that he can't get out of mom, believe me, he will use this leverage to make his life more fun, but it's likely to drive a wedge between you and your partner. You need to be always on the same page so that there is no doubt in the toddler's mind that he has the upper hand.

The worry of leaving toddler with others

This can become a huge weight on your shoulders if you allow it to become one. The best way to arrange for a babysitter or for your parents to get involved with the toddler is to have a very established routine and to make sure that all people who will care for the child adhere to it. Explain the necessity of regular bedtimes. Talk about what is acceptable and what is not acceptable, because the problem here is that when people step into a new routine, it can be very hard for parents to get the child back to the original routine when the child comes home.

Write out a schedule and unless you are certain that those looking after the child will stick to it, find alternatives.

One of the biggest bugbears to the relationship is the fact that baby gets all of the attention. Therefore, it's important for couples to spend enough time with one another and to carry on the relationship even though baby is also part of it now. Sharing the growing up pains and joys is something that's very special indeed and you can keep in touch these days by text or even by Skype when you are absent from one another. Remember, just because you are stuck at home with a toddler doesn't mean that you cannot claim time for yourself. If you want exercise classes, why not time them in with the afternoon nap? If you want to continue to work from home, as long as you can separate things in your life in a reasonable way, there's no reason why you cannot achieve this. You just need to remember that the child does come first because the child needs guidance. However, if you organize your home in such a way that you are able to look over your child while you work, then you may be able to find a good balance and be able to continue working and contributing financially to the relationship. This takes a little pressure off your partner and means that he will be able to spend more time at home with you enjoying watching your child grow up.

You need social interaction. You also need to feel that you have friends so don't make the mistake of giving up contact with friends just because you have a toddler. Okay, those friends may not be into toddler talk, but you can trade evenings with your partner, so that you each get time with your friends as well as being homebound parents. That way, you retain the balance and are a happier and more balanced parent for your child. A parent who begrudges giving up her life to motherhood often carries a lot of bitterness with her and you may not think so now, but kids can pick up on this. It also doesn't help the dynamics of the relationship if you harbor resentment, rather than adjusting your lives to suit both you and your child.

Of all of the toddlers that I looked after during times of crisis, I remember those that came from couples who were actually happy together as being the easiest children to put to bed at night. That's because in their little minds, they harbored no doubts about who mommy and daddy were or the role that they played in their lives. Even though these were foster kids, I can tell you that their lives were defined by who they knew their parents to be and if the parents loved each other and loved their child, the child managed to sleep much better than those poor kids whose parents were unhappy and in the process of separation. The happier you are, the happier your kid will be, so celebrate life and let your toddler see you as a happy and fulfilled human being he/she can respect and love as well as rely upon for positive feedback and learning.

Conclusion

You may have read this far but not yet practiced the different aspects of putting a young toddler to bed. It's a good thing to be prepared and I would suggest that you go back through all of the chapters and use them to approach the topic correctly. These are proven methods and they have also used my experience because there's nothing worse than finding you don't have the means to do what you need to do when emergencies happen. For example, it wakes the whole household if you have to go in search of diapers in the middle of the night, when in fact these could have been stored in a cabinet near the bed so that you can access them easily. It's also a good idea to have a waste disposal bin where you can placed soiled diapers and where they are hygienically placed until you have time the next day to dispose of them. If you are lucky enough to have a bathroom near the child's room, this is useful for this purpose and gives you the added benefit of being able to simply change the diaper and not let the whole process wake you and the child up from an otherwise peaceful night.

If you prepare the nursery for the child and for all eventualities, it makes life so much easier, but remember that there are certain items that must be kept under lock and key or at least out of reach of the child so that there is no danger presented to the child. Creams and lotions, medications and other items should be locked away at all times because there's nothing more tempting to a bored child than to lick something that smells good.

You are going to find that different children react in different ways and that's to be expected. Girls, as stated above, tend to transition to the bedtime routine better than boys do. If you have boys and girls, then watch out for fierce competition between them for mama's attention. If you find that this becomes a problem start to change the night time routine so that each child contributes. For example, one may choose the reading material. One may decide who's going to tell the story tonight, but try to make the whole scenario not about the individual child but about the family as a whole. That way, the child does not feel left out in any of the stages of bedtime training. When it comes to serving up the supper to multiple children, treat them all in the same way and make sure that one does not get more than the other because arguments at this time of the day do not work well toward peaceful routines. If a child feels left out for some reason, he may act up and bedtime is not a time when you want this to happen.

With toddlers, you can get away with bathing several toddlers in the same bath, making this area of the preparation a little easier to handle. I was once watching a couple that had triplets going into action preparing their kids for bed and it was like clockwork. The kids knew what to expect and they didn't fight it because it made logical sense of their lives among their siblings. There were no favorites and every child was treated in exactly the same manner, making it easy for the children to understand that the bedtime routine applied to them all. A child can become difficult at bedtime, but they are testing the waters to a certain extent. When you let the child know that bedtime is non-negotiable, it makes the whole thing easier. If they want to watch something on TV and it falls after their bedtime, record it and let them watch it the next day, but if you break the rules for them one night and let them stay up, you are heading for disaster because their minds will already have established that they can get away with changing your mind and that all they have to do is play up a little to get what they want.

Sometimes singing at bedtime works better than stories and if this is the case, then try it out and choose songs that are not disruptive or that require them to do any action other than sleep. Lullabies are good and children love to look back on their younger years and remember a lullaby that reminds them of mom. However, remember that the song should be a peaceful and calm one as that's the atmosphere that you are trying to create.

I hope that this book has been of help to you and if there are any areas of doubt left, then you need to reread because it is comprehensive in its coverage of all of the aspects you need to take into account when putting little ones to bed. I have purposely covered the situation, from establishing a routine, right through to easy-to-follow steps, but I have also remembered to include the importance to parents that they too get sufficient sleep. You cannot care for boisterous kids when you have no energy yourself. Thus show your kids by example that sleeping isn't a punishment, but that in fact it's a pleasurable thing to do that wakes up all of your energy the next day.

When you go to wake your children in the morning, chances are that they will be awake before you are. However, as toddlers grow so do habits. Some kids will be lazier than others in the morning and you should encourage your child to get up, to get dressed and to come down to breakfast after washing his hands and face, and celebrate this time as family time to look forward to. Sitting down with your kids for breakfast is the best start that you can have to your day and that they can have because it establishes routines that help them to know what to expect out of life. This is a time when children should be told about all the goodness of the food that they are eating and be congratulated for being such good kids. Avoid too much sugar when you are feeding your kids their breakfast as sugar spikes can be exaggerated by the introduction of cereals that are laced with sugar and food additives. Try to provide them with natural nourishment that encourages great digestion and nutrition and you will be able to watch your kids grow healthier and happier, knowing that you have managed to train them to sleep and that they have responded in a very positive manner.

The child who sleeps well is a happy child. He/she is a child who enjoys healthy dreams and happy outcomes. Your contribution to your toddler's happiness and stability will ensure that they get through this stage of their lives with very little in the way of bad memories or insecurity. I have been dealing with the care of toddlers for the past 30 years of my life and every single method mentioned in the book is a potential method to work with your child. With the variety of children I have worked with, I feel that the contents of the book cover all situations and are proven to be effective methods to getting your toddlers off to sleep with the least trauma possible. Just be there for them and let them know they are loved and cared for and the rest will happen all on its own.

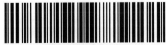

Made in the USA
Columbia, SC
29 April 2019